JUS

Aromatherapy

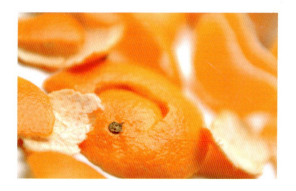

Written and designed by Ark Creative

TOP THAT!™

Contents

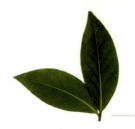

What are

Aromatherapy

Aromatherapy oils, also known as "essential" or "volatile" oils, are the highly fragrant liquid components of aromatic plants, trees, and grasses. They can be found in different parts of the plant including the petals (rose), bark (cinnamon), resin (frankincense), and leaves (eucalyptus).

The term "aromatherapy" dates back to the 1920s when French cosmetic chemist René-Maurice Gattefossé discovered the healing properties of essential oils.

He suffered severe burns to his hand in a laboratory explosion and treated the wound with undiluted lavender essence. It healed without a scar. Essential oils were found to contain powerful antiseptic and painkilling properties.

At that time, Italian doctors, Gatti and Cajola, demonstrated the therapeutic effects of smelling essential oils. The holistic usage of essential oils was further developed in the 1950s when Austrian-born Marguerite Maury introduced the idea of combining them with massage.

Oils?

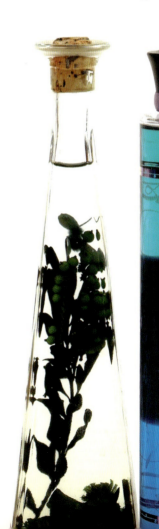

Aromatics 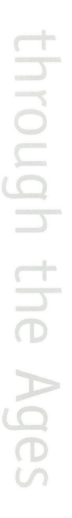 through the Ages

The true founders of aromatherapy are thought to be the ancient Egyptians. They extracted aromatic oils from exotic flowers by squeezing the oil from the petals. The preservative powers of the oils made them an essential part of the embalming process, and they were also blended into perfumes and used as incense.

The Greeks advocated the wearing of fragrant flower garlands and of taking daily aromatic baths, and soon the Romans too were extolling the virtues of healing balms and aromatherapy massage.

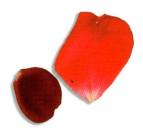

Persian physician Avicenna believed that plant essences strengthened body and spirit, and the Persians developed a passion for the perfume derived from the essential oil of red roses.

In ancient China, alchemists believed that plant extracts contained magical forces to help them develop the elixir of life!

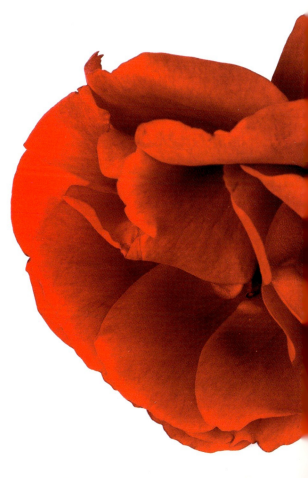

In the

Mood

Knowing a little about the origins of essential oils, you'll be keen to practice the ancient art of aromatherapy for yourself. It's the perfect way to achieve peace of mind—think of it as nature's antidote to stress!

Create your own calming space by using incense sticks or cones to scent your room. Candles complement the theme—especially when they are scented. Specially designed holders should be used for both candles and incense.

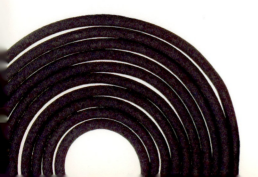

Why not make your own aromatic candle? It's best to buy a chunky beeswax candle to give you the added benefit of honeyed scent! Light it and wait for the wax around the wick to melt. Then blow it out and carefully add a few drops of the essential oil to the molten wax BEFORE relighting.

Warning

Essential oils are highly flammable so NEVER add the oil while the candle is burning.

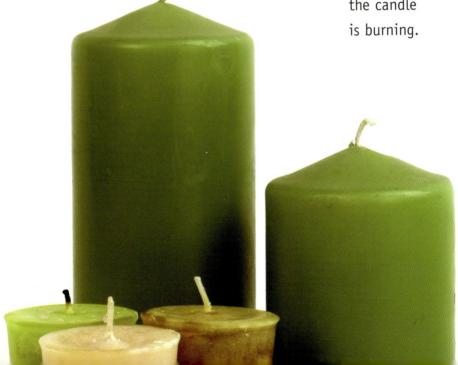

Rest and

Relaxation

At the end of a long day, prepare to kick off your shoes and slide into a warm fragrant bath. This is an excellent way to indulge in essential oils as you'll absorb the oils through your nose and skin.

- ❂ Blend 2 ounces of carrier oil with 20 drops of your favorite-smelling essential oil
- ❂ Store in an amber or cobalt glass bottle
- ❂ Run the bath first (otherwise the vapor will evaporate before you get in)
- ❂ Sprinkle 6 drops of oil onto the water's surface and agitate to disperse well
- ❂ Immerse yourself in heavenly scent!

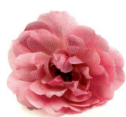

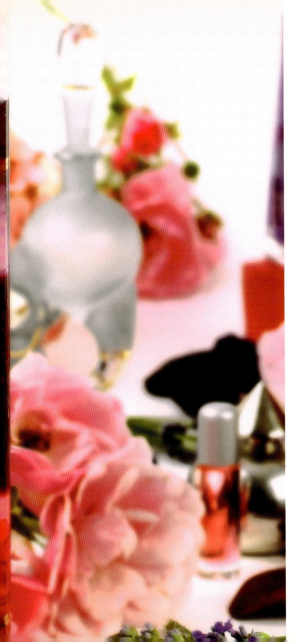

Warning

Essential oils enter the bloodstream through the skin. NEVER apply them directly to your skin as they can be extremely potent. Dilute in a carrier oil and ALWAYS do a patch test first.

Patch test:

- ✿ Mix one drop of the essential oil into a teaspoon of carrier oil
- ✿ Rub a little of the mixture on the inside of your wrist
- ✿ Leave uncovered and unwashed for 24 hours
- ✿ If you suffer no redness or itching the oil is safe to use in a diluted form

Sensual

Calm

Treat your partner to an aromatherapy massage—it will arouse the most primitive senses of smell and touch. Diluted in a carrier oil, then massaged into the skin, essential oils are sure to give the desired spine-tingling effect.

Make your own massage oil by mixing 8-10 drops of skin-friendly essential oil to 1 ounce of carrier oil. Try blending 2 drops of rose otto with 5 drops of sandalwood for a truly sensuous massage.

Tip!

For a superior quality massage, seek "unrefined" carrier oils that still contain their natural vitamins and skin enriching.

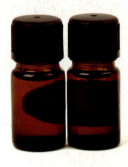

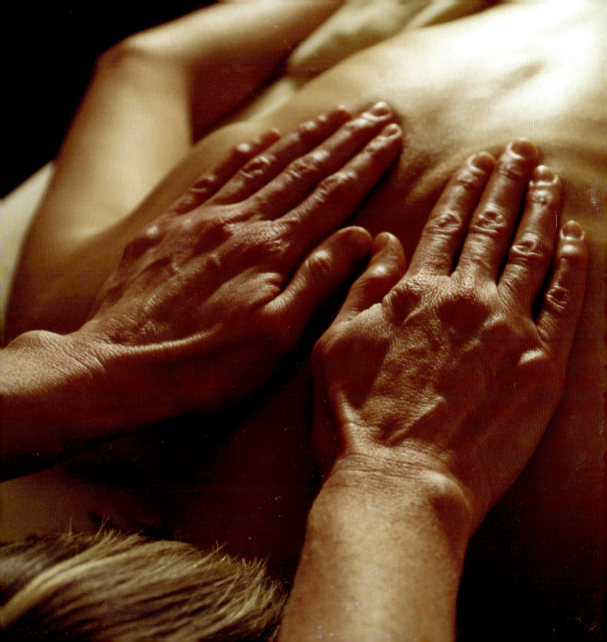

Room

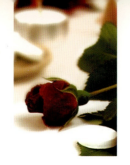

Perfume

Oil burners are a wonderful way to bring harmony into your home.

- ✪ Simply pour some water into the reservoir (this will prevent the oil from heating too quickly)
- ✪ Add some drops of your preferred essential oil
- ✪ Light a candle and place underneath to heat the reservoir
- ✪ As the water heats, the oil will gently warm through and your room will be redolent with gorgeous scent!

Warning

Not all oils sold for use in oil burners are essential. Read the label carefully and follow the manufacturer's instructions for use.

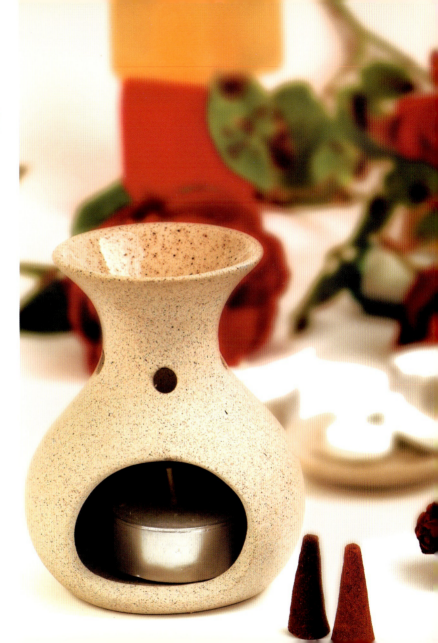

Peaches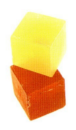

After a bath or shower, your skin is warm and receptive and essential oils will be absorbed quickly. Make the most of it by treating yourself to a homemade massage oil that matches your skin type.

Warning

Remember the potency of these essential oils—patch test your skin before applying and NEVER apply undiluted.

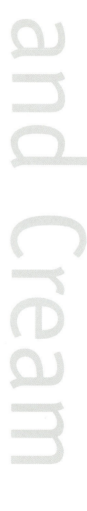

and cream

Normal Skin

Mix 25 ml jojoba oil with 3 drops of lavender and 2 drops of neroli.

Dry Skin

Mix 25 ml peach nut oil with 1 drop of chamomile, 4 drops of lavender, and 10 ml of avocado.

Sensitive Skin

Mix 30 ml almond oil with 1 drop of chamomile.

Oily Skin

Mix 25 ml jojoba oil with 3 drops of cedarwood and 2 drops of frankincense.

NOTE
5ml is equal to 1 teaspoon.
Adjust accordingly.

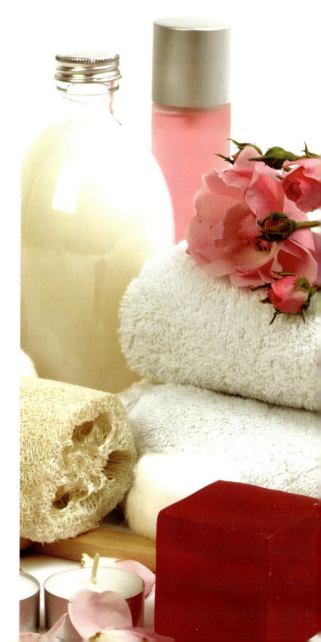

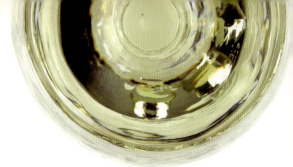

Heady

Scents

Many carrier oils make wonderful conditioning treatments for your hair. Choose from jojoba, peach kernel, and extra virgin olive oil to give your hair a lustrous shine.

Select your hair type from the list opposite and see which essential oils are best suited to you:

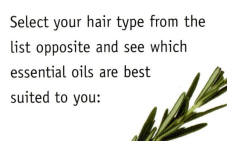

Tip!

Add 2 drops of rosemary or sandalwood to the bristles of your hairbrush and brush through your hair. Heady scents indeed!

Normal Hair

Geranium, lavender, mandarin, neroli, petitgrain, and rose otto

Dry Hair

Chamomile, sandalwood, jojoba, and ylang ylang

Fine Hair

Patchouli and rosemary

Greasy Hair

Eucalyptus, grapefruit, lemon, tea tree, and cypress

19

Bed of Roses

The seductive power

of scent and the way in which it lifts our spirits is rooted deep within us—whether it's the smell of newly mown grass, the mouth-watering smell of baking in the kitchen, or the crisp clean fragrance of fresh laundry.

Bring a woody fragrance to your laundry by adding some drops of frankincense or sandalwood to the distilled water in your steam iron.

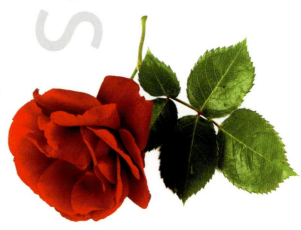

For restful sleep and sweet dreams mix 15 drops of rose otto or lavender oil to 125 ml of water and spray over your bed linen.

Keep drawers fresh by lining them with wallpaper that has first been cut to size and sprayed with a strong aromatic concentrate of your chosen essential oil (40 drops to 50 ml of water).

Tip!

If you have an open fire, perfume the room by burning aromatic plants such as lavender flowers and rosemary twigs.

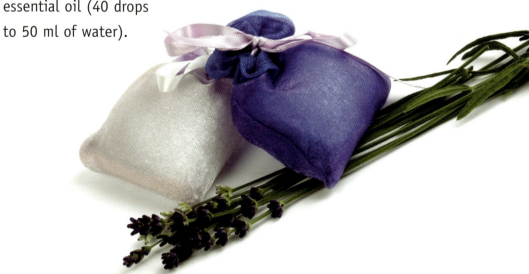

Music to your Senses

Perfume notes were the creation of nineteenth century French perfumer Charles Piesse. He categorized the aroma of essential oils to relate to a scale of top, middle, and base notes, like those of a musical stave.

The perfume industry still uses these three categories today—a good blend of perfume is a well-balanced combination of top, middle, and base notes.

Tip!

Base notes "fix" the fragrance and make it last longer.

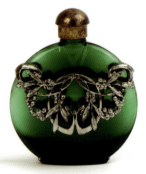

In aromatherapy, the top (head) notes are the most volatile essential oils because they are fast acting and evaporate quickly. Middle (heart) notes are therapeutic and balancing, and base (bottom) notes are the least volatile oils that have a long-lasting effect.

Stimulating your senses, the top note is what you smell first. This fades away leaving you with the heart note and when this too fades, you can still smell the bottom note which lingers long after the other two have gone.

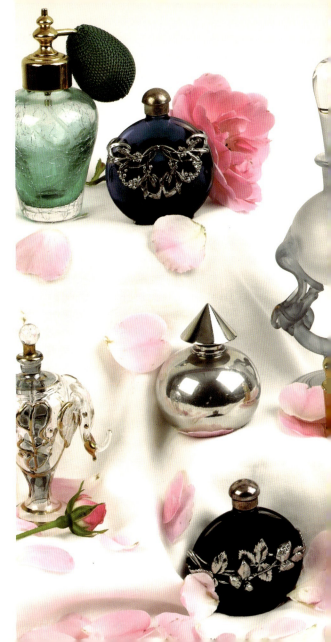

Harmonizing

Have a go at composing your own perfumes by experimenting with different blends of aromatic notes. Some scents stand out as popular solo artists on their own and you may not want to blend these with anything at all. Rose otto, ylang ylang, jasmine, and patchouli are the most common of these.

With so many oils to choose from, it's helpful to know that essences can be categorized into their own musical "family" and that as a rule, aromatic notes from the same family harmonize well together.

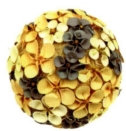

Tip!

The Victorian era popularized the use of essential oils as a tonic to lift the spirits. You too can benefit by adapting their recipe for smelling salts—just mix a few drops of your favorite scented oil with some rock salt. Orange and patchouli is the perfect pick-me-up!

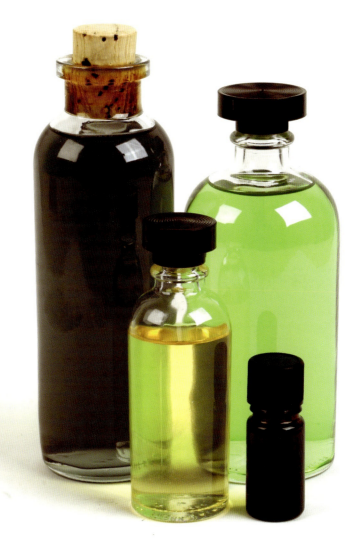

A Symphony of

Start creating your symphony by selecting 2-4 drops of essential oils from the same family, then dilute them in 10 ml of carrier oil.

THE AROMATIC FAMILY

CITRUS	FLORAL	HERBACEOUS	* CAMPHORACEOUS
grapefruit	geranium	chamomile	eucalyptus
lemon	chamomile	lavender	rosemary
lime	rose otto	peppermint	peppermint
mandarin	lavender	rosemary	tea tree
orange	ylang ylang	marjoram	lavender
	neroli	clary sage	

Scents

	SPICY	RESINOUS	WOODY	EARTHY
	black pepper	frankincense	cedarwood	patchouli
	ginger	myrrh	sandalwood	vetiver
			juniper	
			cypress	

* Camphoraceous aromatics are medicinal and contain counterirritant, healing and antiseptic properties. They may also be used in the treatment of colds.

Carrier Oils

Carrier oils (sometimes called vegetable, base, or fixed oils) are derived from the fatty portions of seeds, nuts, vegetables, and plants. These are the base oils used to dilute essential oils before applying them to the skin, so called because they "carry" the essential oil onto your skin.

Carrier oils do not evaporate when heated, neither do they impart their aroma as strongly as essential oils. For this reason always try to obtain "cold pressed" or "extra virgin" carrier oils as these will contain the most therapeutic properties.

Originating from the fatty portions of plants means that all carrier oils make excellent choices for massage as they are rich in nutrients and moisturizing properties.

Tip!

Purchase carrier oils in small quantities as their shelf life is only three months.

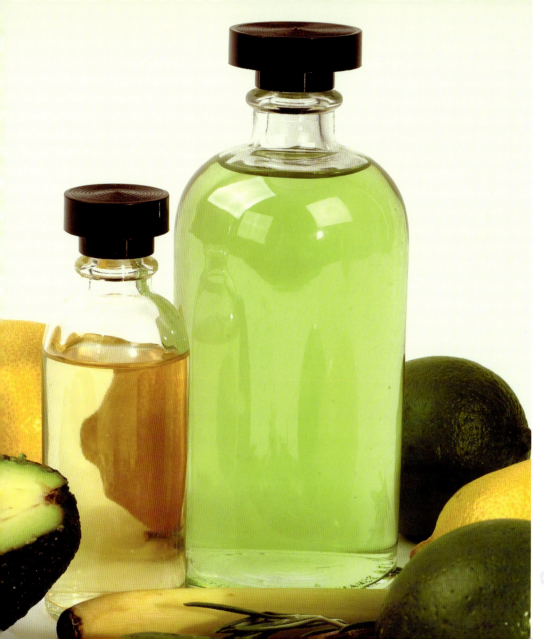

Apricot Kernel

Apricot Kernel

Plant: Apricot Kernel

Botanical name: Prunus armeniaca

Origins: Extracted from the seed kernel of the fruit.

Aroma: Faint smell of marzipan.

Properties: Light textured, easily absorbed, contains vitamins A and C.

Uses: A special oil used mainly in beauty care, and an excellent base for a face or body massage.

Apricot Kernel

Avocado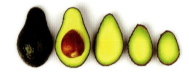

Plant: Avocado

Botanical name: Persea americana

Origins: Best quality is cold pressed from the flesh of the fruit.

Aroma: Faintly nutty.

Properties: Highly penetrative, rich in essential fatty acids, betacarotene, and vitamin E.

Uses: A special oil used mainly in beauty care— excellent for dry, aging skin, or skin dehydrated by too much sunbathing!

Avocado

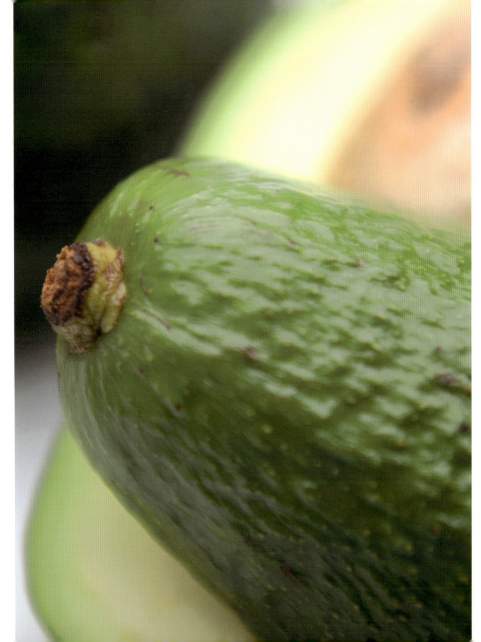

Avocado

Borage

Plant: Borage

Botanical name: Borago officinalis

Origins: Warm pressed or solvent extracted from the tiny seeds of the beautiful blue starflower plant —is often labeled "Starflower" for this reason.

Aroma: Light and sweet.

Properties: Rich source of essential fatty acids.

Uses: A special oil used mainly in beauty care. The best way to enhance your skin is to take "Starflower" capsules as a nutritional supplement.

Borage

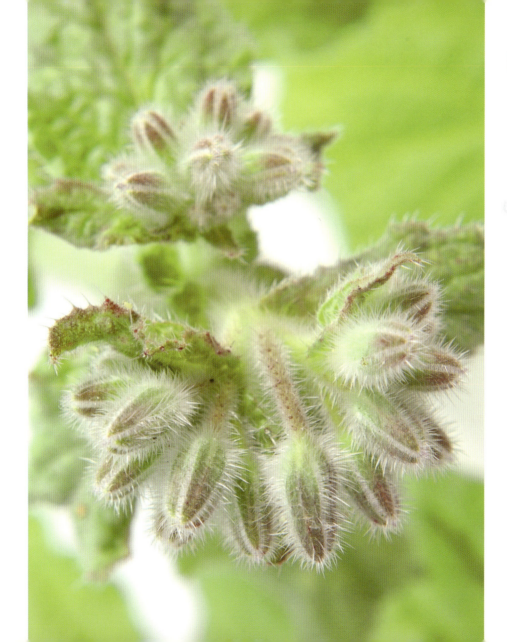

Borage

Evening Primrose

Plant: Evening Primrose

Botanical name: Oenothera biennis

Origins: Extracted from the tiny seeds of the bright yellow flowers which bloom only at night.

Aroma: Faint and musty.

Properties: Contains vitamins, minerals, and essential fatty acids.

Uses: A nutritional supplement to treat premenstrual syndrome, period pains, arthritis, and rheumatism. It is also excellent as a moisturizing beauty treatment.

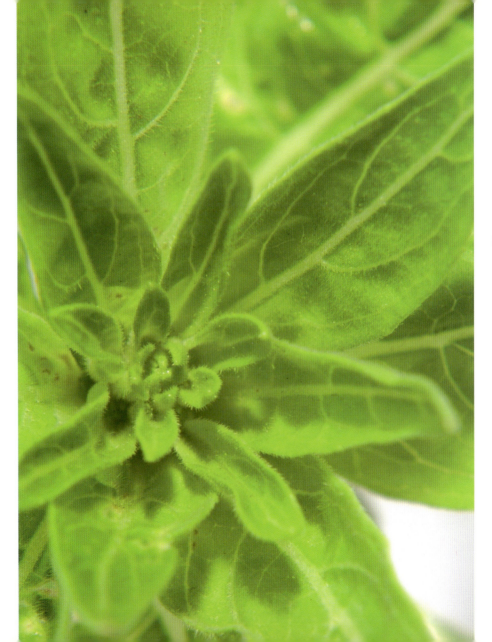

Evening Primrose

Grapeseed

Plant: Grapeseed

Botanical name: Vitis vinifera

Origins: Heat extracted from the seeds of the fruit.

Aroma: Hardly any.

Properties: Heat extraction destroys the nutrients.

Uses: This is a popular massage oil.

Grapeseed

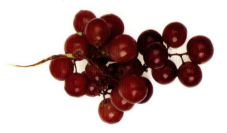

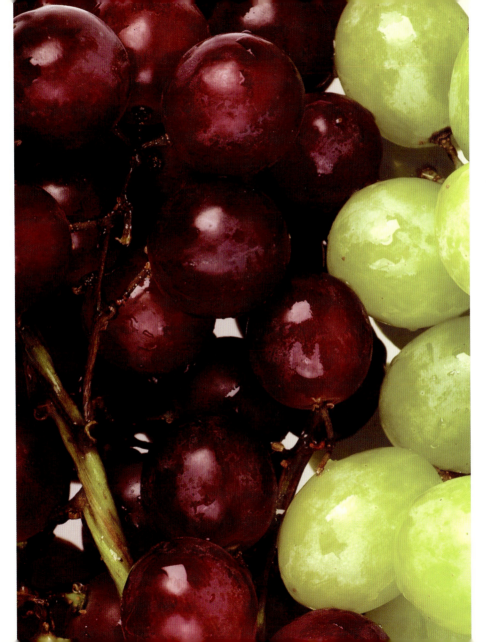

Grapeseed

Jojoba

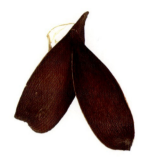

Plant: Jojoba

Botanical name: Simmondsia chinensis

Origins: Liquid wax extracted from the beans of the plant.

Aroma: Hardly any.

Properties: Highly penetrative, also has some anti-inflammatory properties.

Uses: A special oil used mainly in beauty care. It is an excellent moisturizer for all skin types, and makes a good conditioning treatment for dry hair.

Jojoba

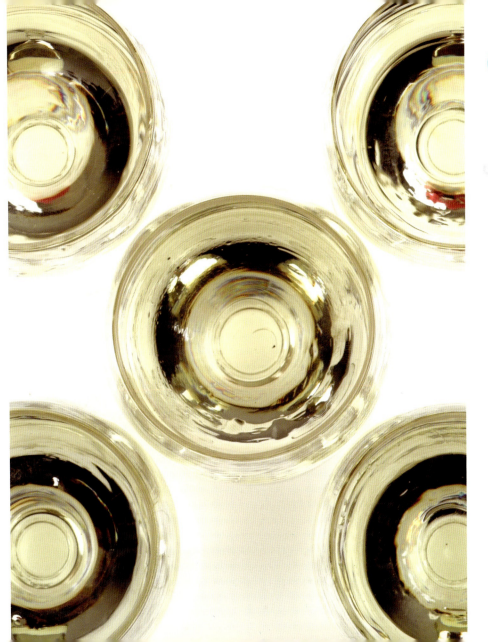

Jojoba

Peach Kernel

Peach Kernel

Plant: Peach Kernel

Botanical name: Prunus persica

Origins: Best quality is cold pressed from the kernels of the fruit.

Aroma: Delicate peachy aroma.

Properties: Fine textured so easily absorbed into the skin.

Uses: A special oil used mainly in beauty care, peach kernel oil is ideal for facial massage since it's kind to the skin. It will also add shine to hair.

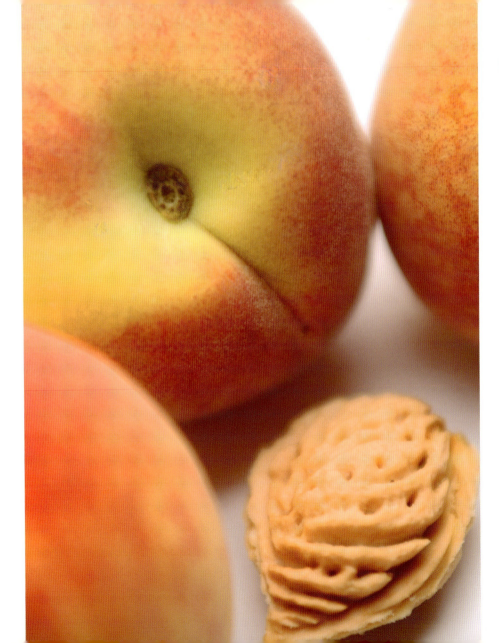

Peach Kernel

Sweet Almond

Plant: Sweet Almond

Botanical name: Prunus dulcis

Origins: Extracted from the kernels of the sweet almond tree.

Aroma: Faint nutty scent.

Properties: Contains vitamins D and E, also has some anti-inflammatory properties.

Uses: It is excellent for treating psoriasis, eczema and dermatitis—or to relieve sunburn.

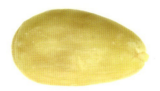

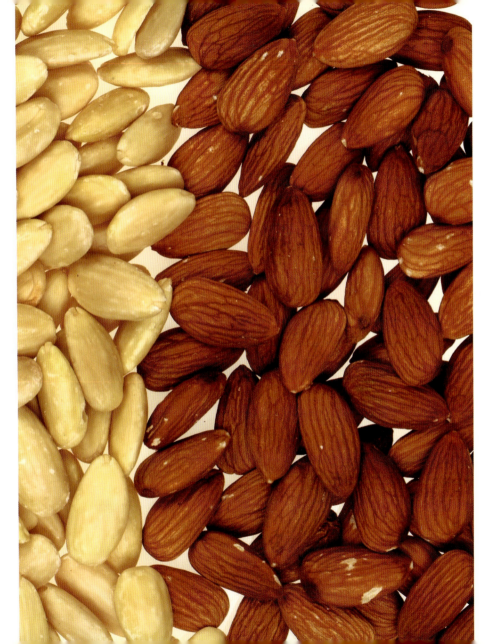

Sweet Almond

Infused Oils

Infused oils, sometimes called "macerated" oils, are commercially made when the amount of essential oil in the plant is very small and therefore expensive to extract. Fresh plant matter is soaked or "macerated" in a high quality carrier oil so that the essential oils are dissolved and impart their fragrance.

Plant: Hypericum (or St John's Wort)

Botanical name: Hypericum perforatum

Part used: Leaves and flowers.

Properties: Anti-inflammatory, anti-rheumatic.

Uses: It will ease rheumatism, sciatica, sunburn and bruises.

Plant: Calendula (or marigold)

Botanical name: Calendula officinalis

Part used: Flowers

Properties: Anti-inflammatory, antifungal.

Uses: This is excellent for treating eczema and diaper rash and soothes sore, inflamed and itchy skin.

Infused Oils

Top 20 Essential Oils

Now you know what constitutes a carrier oil and what is meant by an infused oil, you're ready to try your hand at blending and experimenting with some aromatic oils of your choice! Take your pick from the "Top 20" we've selected for you. Don't forget to try composing some subtle harmonies of your own by blending some top, middle and base notes together to compose a fragrant signature.

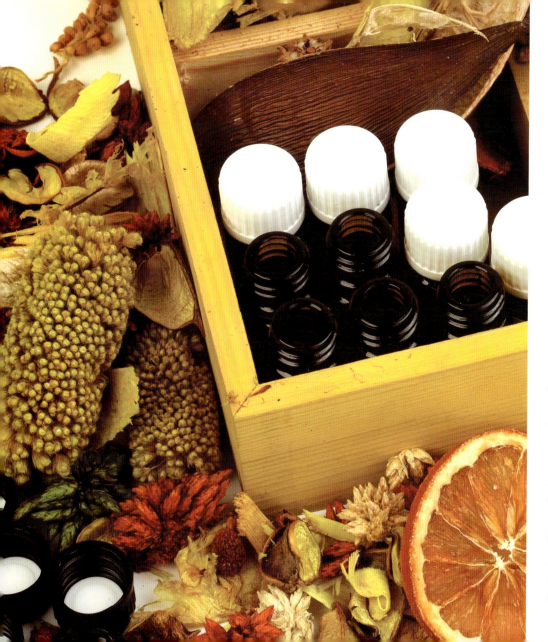

Chamomile

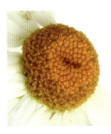

number 1

Plant: Chamomile

Botanical name: Anthemis nobilis

Origins: Extracted from the flower heads.

Aroma: Sweet and fruity.

Properties: Anti-inflammatory and antiseptic.

Uses: A good treatment for premenstrual syndrome, insect bites, stings, insomnia, and eczema.

Suggested Blends: Lavender, geranium, jasmine, rose otto, and neroli.

Perfume Note: Middle

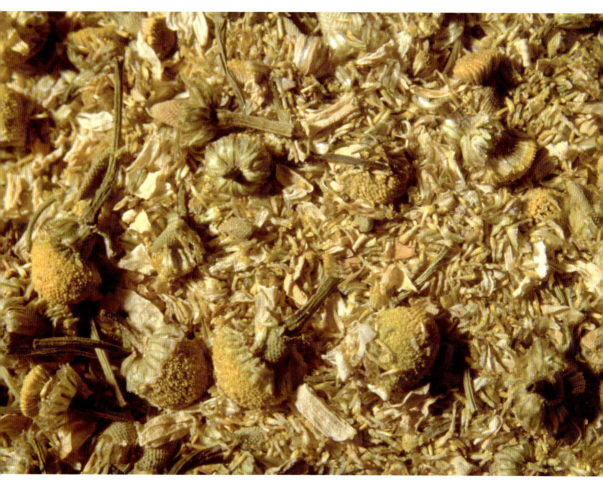

Cedarwood Atlas

number 2

Plant: Cedarwood Atlas

Botanical name: Anthemis nobilis

Origins: Distilled from the wood shavings and sawdust.

Aroma: Sweet and woody.

Properties: Antiseptic, astringent, and sedative.

Uses: A good treatment for cystitis, fungal infections, dandruff, insect bites, and stings.

Suggested Blends: Frankincense, ylang ylang, vetiver, juniper, and rosemary.

Perfume Note: Base

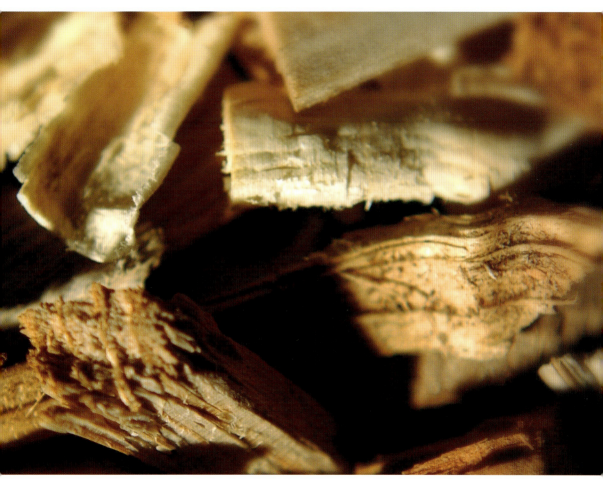

Clary Sage

WARNING!
Do NOT use
if you are
pregnant.

number 3

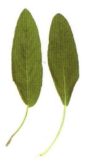

Plant: Clary Sage

Botanical name: Salvia sclarea

Origins: Distilled from the leaves and flower tops.

Aroma: Fruity and flowery.

Properties: Antidepressant, sedative, and anti-inflammatory.

Uses: Clary sage can reduce high blood pressure, and ease depression, nervous tension, and stress.

Suggested Blends: Lavender, tea tree, and sandalwood.

Perfume Note: Middle

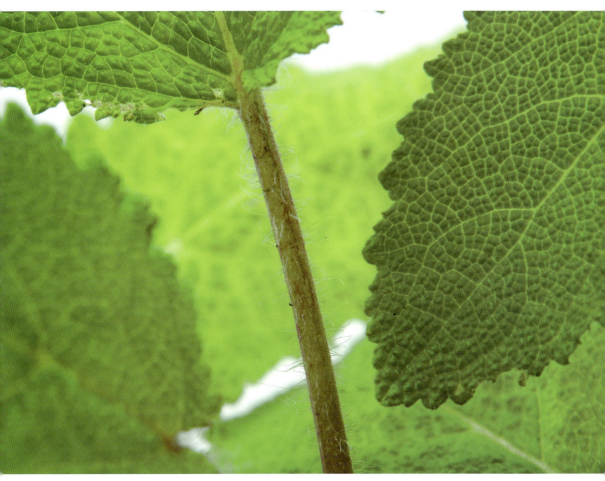

Cypress

Plant: Cypress

Botanical name: Cupressus sempervirens

Origins: Distilled from the needles and twigs of young branches.

Aroma: Soft, piney, and woody.

Properties: Astringent, antiseptic, and antispasmodic.

Uses: This is valuable for treating varicose veins, menstruation, and menopausal problems.

Suggested Blends: Clary sage, frankincense, juniper, and lemongrass.

Perfume Note: Middle

Eucalyptus

Plant: Eucalyptus

Botanical name: Eucalyptus globulus

Origins: Distilled from the leaves and young twigs.

Aroma: Strong camphoraceous (medicinal) smell.

Properties: Antiseptic, anti rheumatic, and analgesic.

Uses: Nature's first aid treatment for cuts, bruises and blisters. It is also excellent for coughs, colds, throat infections, and congestion.

Suggested Blends: Lavender, tea tree, sandalwood, and rosemary.

Perfume Note: Top

WARNING! NEVER take orally as it is very toxic.

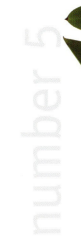

Frankincense

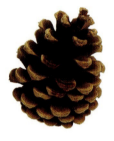

number 6

Plant: Frankincense

Botanical name: Boswellia carterii

Origins: Extracted from the gum resin which collects when incisions are made into the bark.

Aroma: Warm and piney, with a hint of camphor.

Properties: Astringent, antiseptic, and sedative.

Uses: A good treatment for abscesses, ulcers, asthma, and bronchitis.

Suggested Blends: Grapefruit, patchouli, rose otto, and juniper.

Perfume Note: Base

number 6

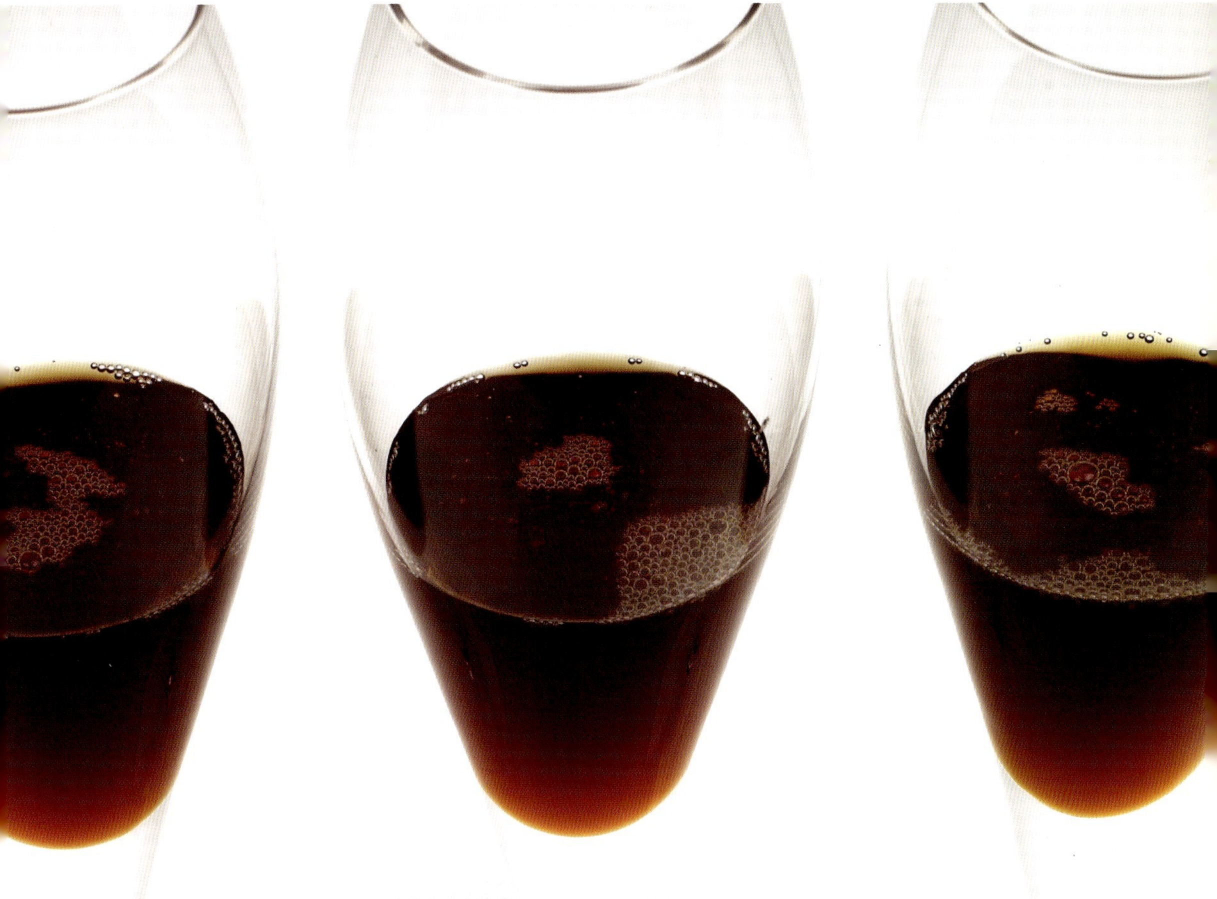

Geranium

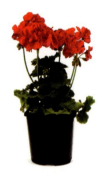

number 7

Plant: Geranium

Botanical name: Pelargonium odoratissimum

Origins: Distilled from the leaves, stalks, and flowers

Aroma: Rose-scented, sweet, and heavy.

Properties: Analgesic, antiseptic, and astringent.

Uses: An excellent treatment for premenstrual syndrome, stress, cuts, and skin problems.

Suggested Blends: Grapefruit, orange, lavender, and neroli.

Perfume Note: Middle

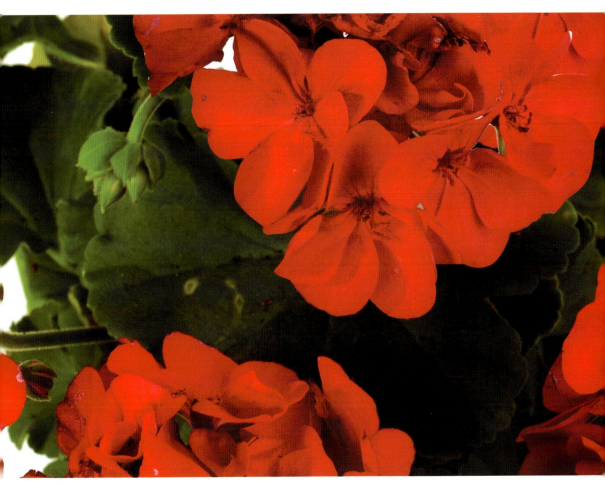

Grapefruit

number 8

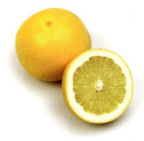

Plant: Grapefruit

Botanical name: Citrus paradisi odoratissimum

Origins: Extracted from the fresh fruit peel.

Aroma: Clean, sharp citrus tang.

Properties: Digestive, antiseptic, and astringent.

Uses: A good treatment for oily skin, acne, and cellulite.

Suggested Blends: Orange, tangerine, peppermint, and neroli.

Perfume Note: Top

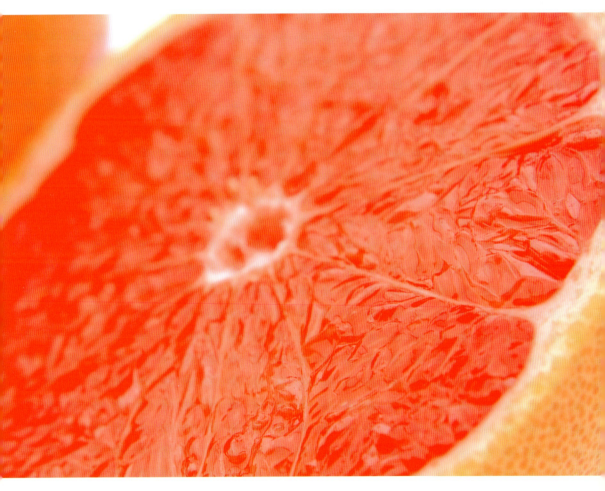

Lavender

Plant: Lavender

Botanical name: Lavandula augustifolia

Origins: Distilled from the flowering shrub tips.

Aroma: Sweet, flowery, and herbaceous.

Properties: Analgesic, sedative, and antiseptic.

Uses: Nature's first aid treatment for burns because it accelerates cell growth and repair. It has remarkable healing properties and can be used to alleviate high blood pressure and stress.

Suggested Blends: Rose otto, geranium, patchouli, rosemary, and frankincense.

Perfume Note: Top/Middle

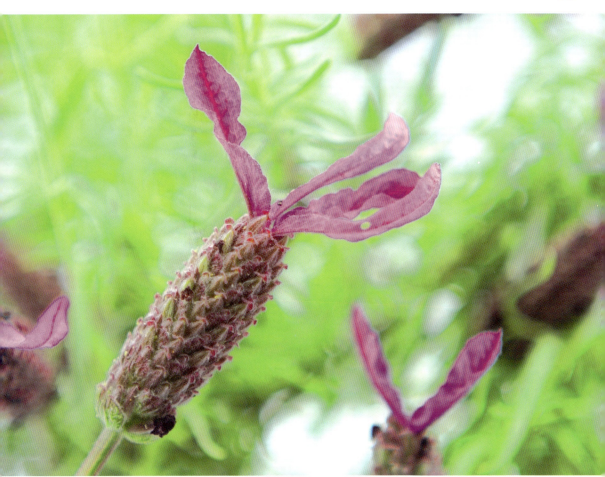

Lemon

number 10

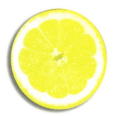

Plant: Lemon

Botanical name: Citrus limon

Origins: Extracted from the peel of the fruit.

Aroma: Fresh and sharp.

Properties: Insecticidal, astringent, and anti-rheumatic.

Uses: Excellent for oily skin, brittle nails, arthritis, and rheumatism.

Suggested Blends: Chamomile, tangerine, juniper, myrrh, and petitgrain.

Perfume Note: Top

CAUTION! Lemon oil only keeps for about six months.

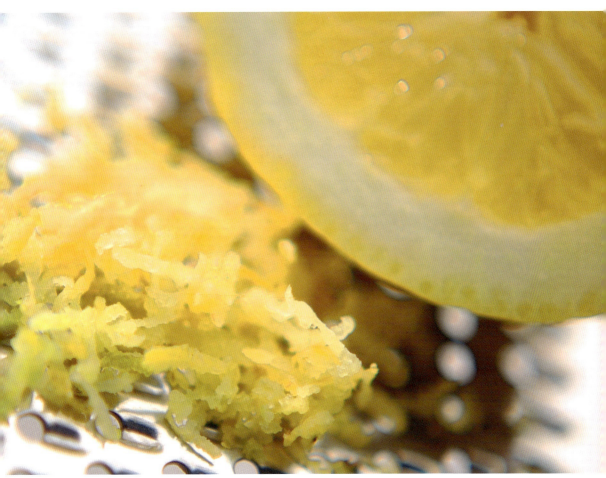

Lime

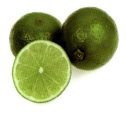

Plant: Lime

Botanical name: Citrus aurantifolia

Origins: Extracted from the peel of the fruit.

Aroma: Bright, fresh, and citrus.

Properties: Antiseptic and restorative.

Uses: To treat colds, depression, and stress.

Suggested Blends:
Lavender, rosemary, grapefruit, and orange.

Perfume Note: Top

CAUTION!
Lime oil only keeps for about six months.

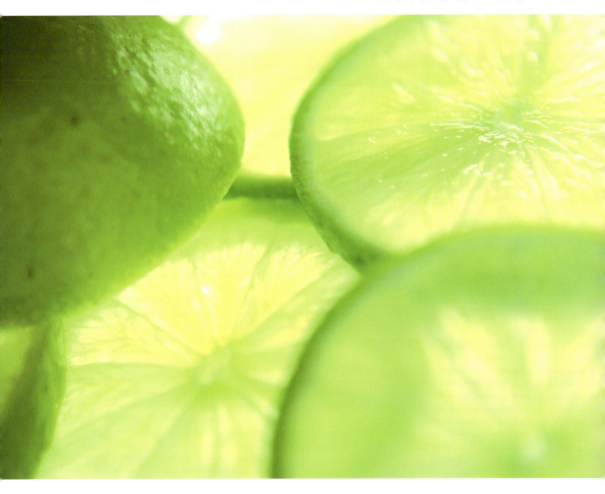

Mandarin

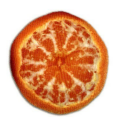

Plant: Mandarin

Botanical name: Citrus nobilis

Origins: Extracted from the peel of the fruit.

Aroma: Sweet and citrus.

Properties: Digestive, laxative, and sedative.

Uses: This is good for children's problems such as colic, hiccups, and coughs. It will also help to prevent stretch marks during pregnancy.

Suggested Blends: Lemongrass, rose otto, lemon, and grapefruit.

Perfume Note: Top

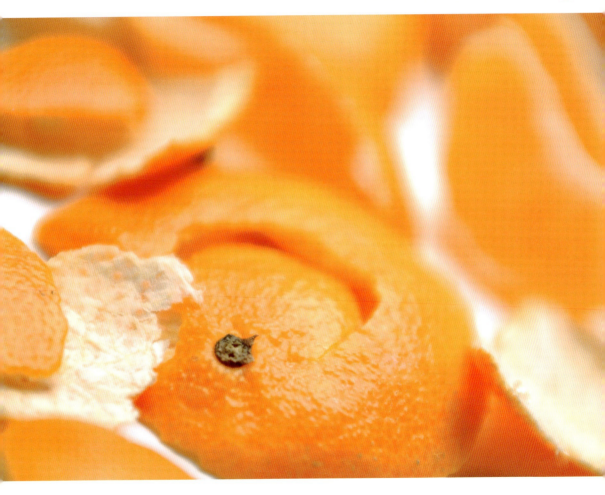

Neroli

number 13

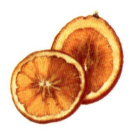

Plant: Neroli

Botanical name: Citrus aurantium

Origins: Distilled from the blossom of the orange tree.

Aroma: Sweet and floral.

Properties: Antidepressant and antiseptic. It's also reputed to be an aphrodisiac!

Uses: An excellent remedy for stress, skin care, and heart palpitations.

Suggested Blends: Ginger, jasmine, lavender, and orange.

Perfume Note: Middle

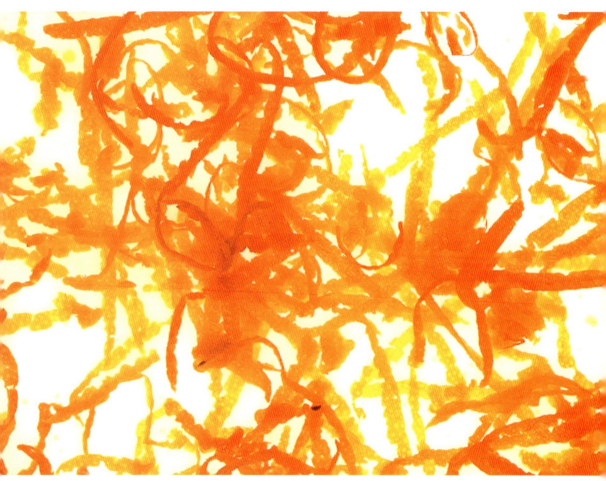

Orange

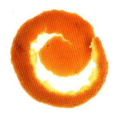

number 14

Plant: Orange

Botanical name: Citrus sinensis

Origins: Extracted from the peel of the fruit.

Aroma: Deliciously orangy.

Properties: Antidepressant and a tonic.

Uses: Will balance the digestive system and helps to lower blood pressure.

Suggested Blends: Clary sage, lavender, and ginger.

Perfume Note: Top

CAUTION! Orange oil only keeps for about six months.

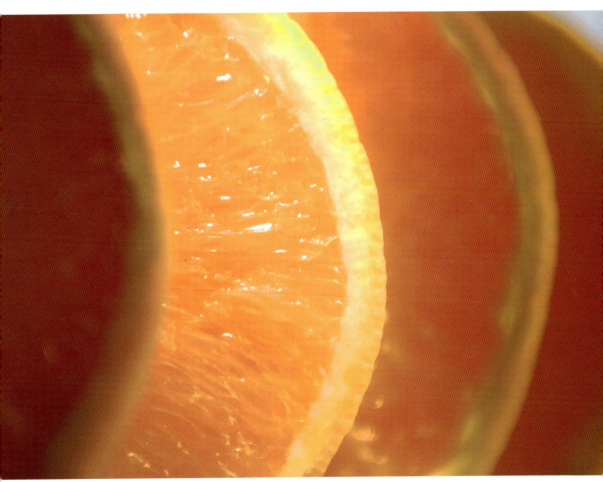

Peppermint

number 15

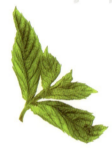

WARNING!
Do NOT use
if you are
pregnant.

Plant: Peppermint

Botanical name: Mentha piperita

Origins: Distilled from the flower tops.

Aroma: Mint-scented and fresh.

Properties: Anti-inflammatory, antiseptic, and digestive.

Uses: It's excellent for indigestion, nausea, diarrhea, colitis, and sinus congestion. Will also make a good mosquito repellent.

Suggested Blends: Rosemary, lavender, eucalyptus, and lemon.

Perfume Note: Top

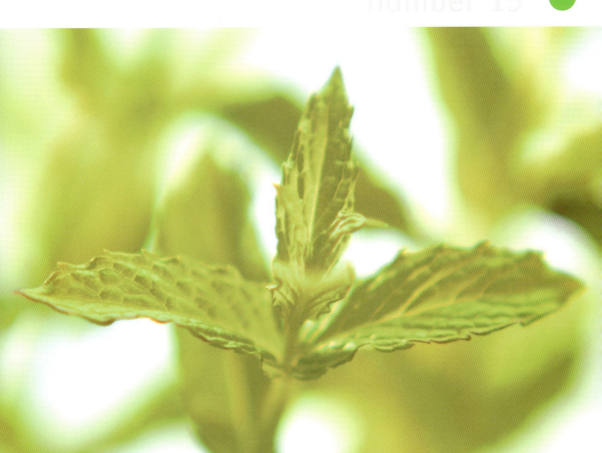

Rose Otto

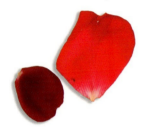

number 16

Plant: Rose Otto

Botanical name: Rosa damascena

Origins: Distilled from the fresh rose petals.

Aroma: Sweet, with a hint of vanilla.

Properties: Sedative, antidepressant, and a tonic.

Uses: Rosewater is a popular skin tonic. It is also used to combat menstrual disorders and stress.

Suggested Blends: Ylang ylang, geranium, patchouli, chamomile, and frankincense.

Perfume Note: Middle to top

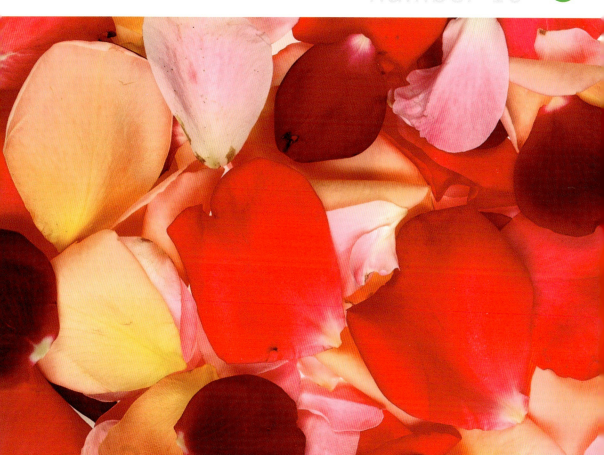

Rosemary

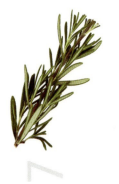

WARNING!
Do NOT use if you are either pregnant or epileptic.

Plant: Rosemary

Botanical name:
Rosmarinus officinalis

Origins: Steam distilled from the flowering tops of the plant.

Aroma: Camphoraceous and balsamic.

Properties: Anti-rheumatic and fungicidal.

Uses: Helps prevent dandruff and adds luster to your hair. Will also ease muscular pain.

Suggested Blends: Tea tree, eucalyptus, geranium, and peppermint.

Perfume Note: Middle

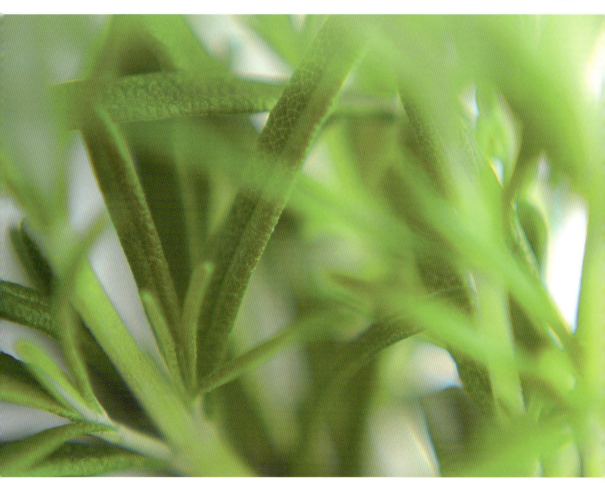

Sandalwood

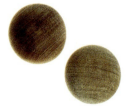

number 18

Plant: Sandalwood

Botanical name: Santalum album

Origins: Distilled from the tree.

Aroma: Soft, sweet, and woody.

Properties: Antiseptic, anti-inflammatory, and antidepressant.

Uses: Used to treat stress, nausea, colic, and catarrh. It is invaluable for dry or inflamed skin.

Suggested Blends: Patchouli, cedarwood, rose otto, bay, and vetiver.

Perfume Note: Base

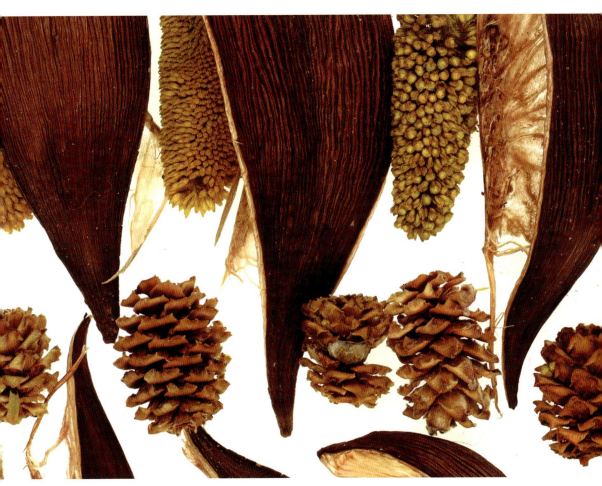

Tea Tree

Plant: Tea Tree

Botanical name: Melaleuca alternifolia

Origins: Distilled from the leaves and twigs of the tree.

Aroma: Strongly medicinal.

Properties: Antibiotic, antiseptic, and fungicidal.

Uses: Nature's first aid for fungal infections such as thrush, athlete's foot. An excellent treatment for mouth ulcers, cold sores, insect bites, and stings.

Suggested Blends: Lavender, rosemary, spearmint, and geranium.

Perfume Note: Middle

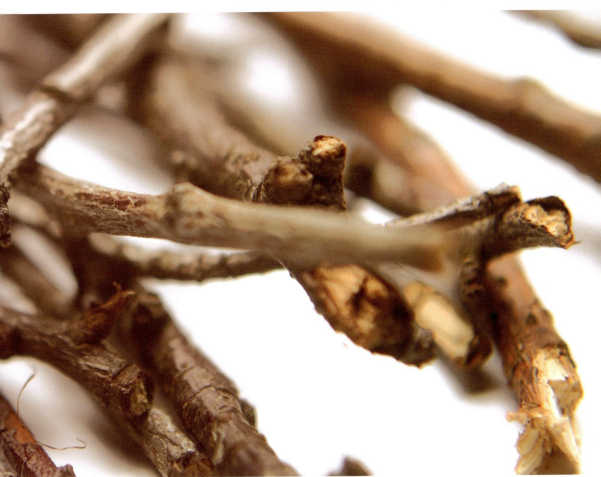

Ylang Ylang

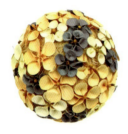

Plant: Ylang Ylang

Botanical name: Cananga odorata

Origins: Steam distilled from the freshly picked flowers.

Aroma: A heady floral mix of almonds and jasmine.

Properties: Sedative, tonic, and antiseptic.

Uses: Used to treat stress, premenstrual syndrome, and nervous tension. A reputed aphrodisiac!

Suggested Blends: Black pepper, lemon, mandarin, grapefruit, and vetiver.

Perfume Note: Base

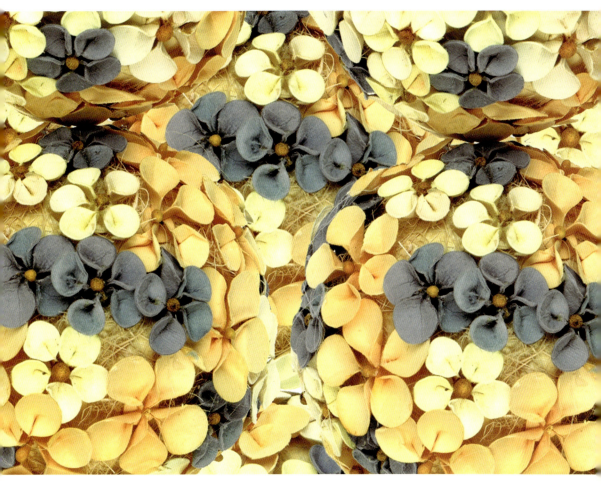

Diffuse your Dreams

Achieving dreamy room fragrances is easy! Your bedroom will be seductively transformed with a hint of any of the following essential oils, which can all be used with a lamp ring.

A lamp ring is a small, circular ring (metal or ceramic) that sits on top of an upward pointing light bulb. A few drops of your preferred aromatic oil can be dropped on to the ring so that the scent evaporates into the room as it heats up.

You could also try using an electric diffuser. This contains an electric heating element to warm a container for your oils, or by passing air from a

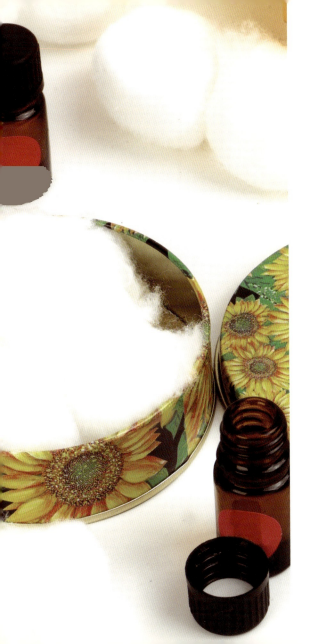

fan through an absorbent pad on to which you have dropped some oil.

Alternatively, why don't you make your own personal diffuser? Drop some oil on to a pad of absorbent cotton, place inside a small tin—make sure the lid has holes in it. Position on a radiator to perfume the room.

Tip!

Lamp rings are NOT recommended for light bulbs stronger than 60 watts.

Basil

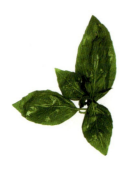

Plant: Basil

Botanical name: Ocimum basilicum

Origins: Steam distilled from the flower tops and leaves.

Aroma: Sweet and herb-scented.

Properties: Antiseptic, restorative, and antidepressant.

Uses: This is good for respiratory problems, anxiety, depression, insect bites, and coughs.

Suggested Blends: Clary sage, frankincense, geranium, and neroli.

Perfume Note: Top

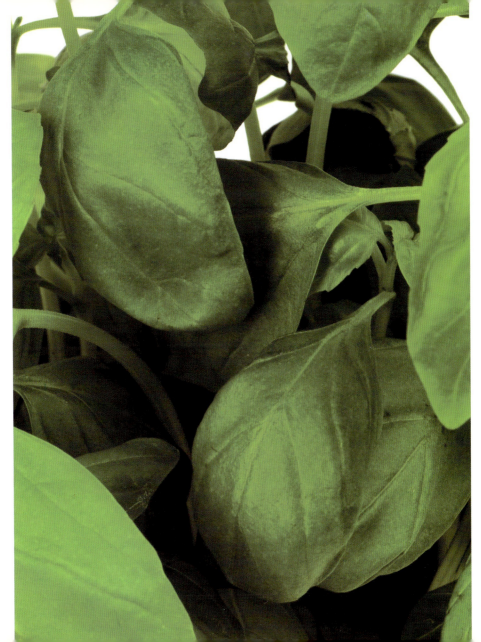

More essential oils

Bay

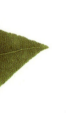

Plant: Bay

Botanical name: Laurus nobilis

Origins: Extracted from the leaves.

Aroma: Spicy and medicinal smelling.

Properties: Restorative and a tonic.

Uses: This is a good treatment for aching muscles, coughs, colds, and rheumatism.

Suggested Blends: Lavender, tea tree, and frankincense.

Perfume Note: Middle

Bay

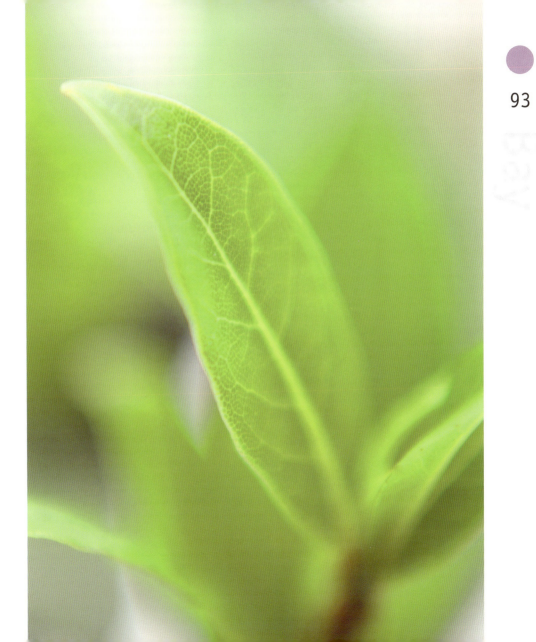

Black Pepper

Plant: Black Pepper

Botanical name: Piper nigrum

Origins: Distilled from the dried black pepper berries (peppercorns).

Aroma: Hot and spicy.

Properties: Appetite stimulant, antiseptic, and digestive.

Uses: An excellent treatment for muscular aches and rheumatism, loss of appetite, and chilblains.

Suggested Blends: Frankincense, sandalwood, lavender, and rosemary.

Perfume Note: Middle

Plant: Citronella

Botanical name: Cymbopogon nardus

Origins: Extracted from the top of the grass.

Aroma: Sharp and lemony.

Properties: Insect repelling and a tonic.

Uses: An excellent scent for your garden candles guaranteed to keep those summer barbecue bugs at bay.

Suggested Blends:
Lavender and rosemary.

Perfume Note: Top

WARNING!
Do NOT use if you are pregnant.

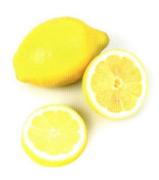

Citronella

Clove Bud

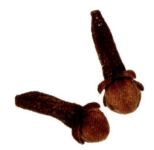

Plant: Clove

Botanical name: Eugenia caryophyllata

Origins: Extracted from the flower buds of the clove tree.

Aroma: Slightly bitter and woody.

WARNING! Do NOT apply directly to skin or inhale via steam applications —best to use as a room scent or fumigant only.

Properties: Antiseptic and anti-rheumatic.

Uses: A classic remedy for toothache, neuralgia, arthritis, and rheumatism. Repels clothes moths.

Suggested Blends: Orange, rose otto, and ylang ylang.

Perfume Note: Middle

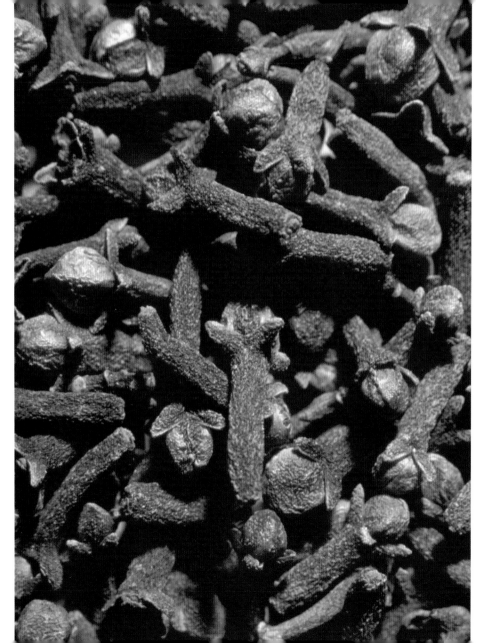

Clove Bud

Fennel

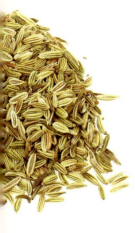

Fennel

Plant: Fennel

Botanical name: Foeniculum vulgare

Origins: Distilled from the crushed seeds.

Aroma: Aniseed

Properties: Anti-inflammatory and a tonic.

Uses: This is used as a tonic for the digestive system and to treat premenstrual problems.

Suggested Blends: Lavender, geranium, and rose otto

Perfume Note: Top/middle

WARNING!
Do NOT use if you are either pregnant or epileptic.

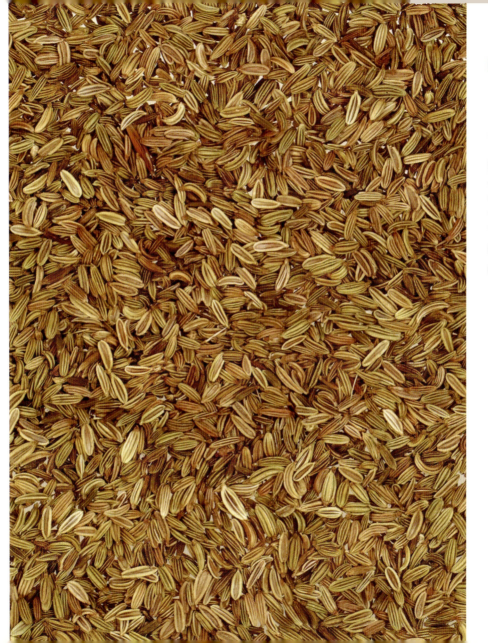

Fennel

Ginger

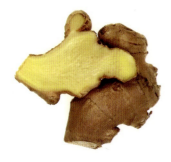

Plant: Ginger

Botanical name: Zingiber officinalis

Origins: Distilled from the dried rhizomes of the plant.

Aroma: Earthy and spicy.

Properties: Antiseptic and stimulant.

Uses: A wonderful remedy for nausea and for catarrh, congestion, and coughs.

Suggested Blends: Grapefuit, geranium, spearmint, and patchouli

Perfume Note: Middle/base

Ginger

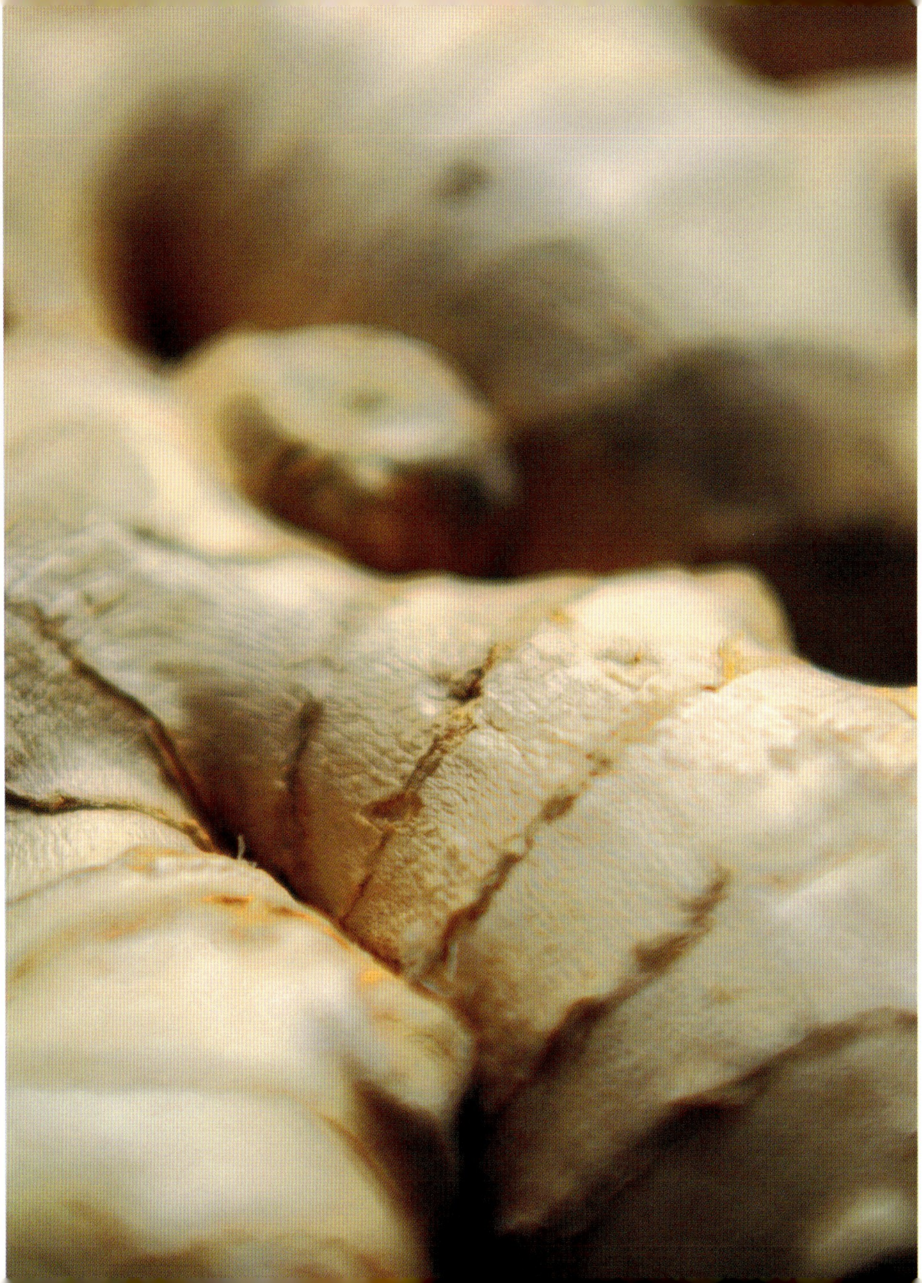

Jasmine

Jasmine

WARNING!
Do NOT use if you are pregnant.

Plant: Jasmine

Botanical name: Jasminum officinalis

Origins: Extracted from flowers picked after dusk when the oil is at its highest concentration.

Aroma: Heady, exotic, and floral.

Properties: Sedative and antidepressant.

Uses: An excellent tonic for labor pains, premenstrual syndrome, and depression.

Suggested Blends: Chamomile, ylang ylang, and sandalwood.

Perfume Note: Middle

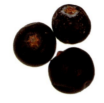

Plant: Juniper

Botanical name: Juniperus communis

Origins: Extracted from the crushed or dried berries.

Aroma: Fresh and woody.

Properties: Antiseptic and sedative.

Uses: This is beneficial in treating skin, arthritis, and rheumatic conditions.

Suggested Blends: Rose otto, clary sage, geranium, grapefruit, and lemon.

Perfume Note: Middle

WARNING!
Do NOT use if you are pregnant.

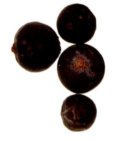

Juniper

Lemongrass

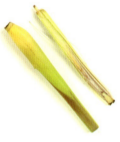

Lemongrass

Plant: Lemongrass

Botanical name: Cymbopogon citratus

Origins: Extracted from the oriental grass.

Aroma: Sweet and lemony.

Properties: Insecticidal, antiseptic, and a tonic.

Uses: This is good for relieving stress and palpitations. It will also stimulate breast milk in nursing mothers.

Suggested Blends: Geranium, myrrh, palmarosa, and petitgrain.

Perfume Note: Top

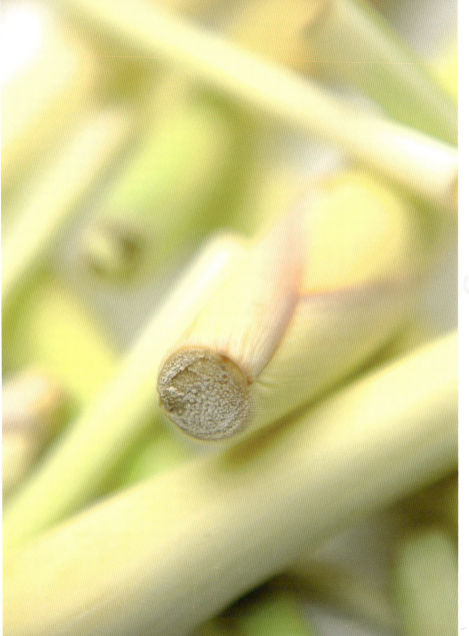

Lemongrass

Marjoram

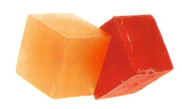

Plant: Marjoram

Botanical name: Origanum marjorana

Origins: Extracted from the leaves.

Aroma: Herbaceous, warm, and spicy.

Properties: Digestive, antiseptic, and sedative.

Uses: It lowers blood pressure, eases muscle injuries and sprains, and aids insomnia.

Suggested Blends: Juniper, tea tree, and rosemary.

Perfume Note: Middle

Marjoram

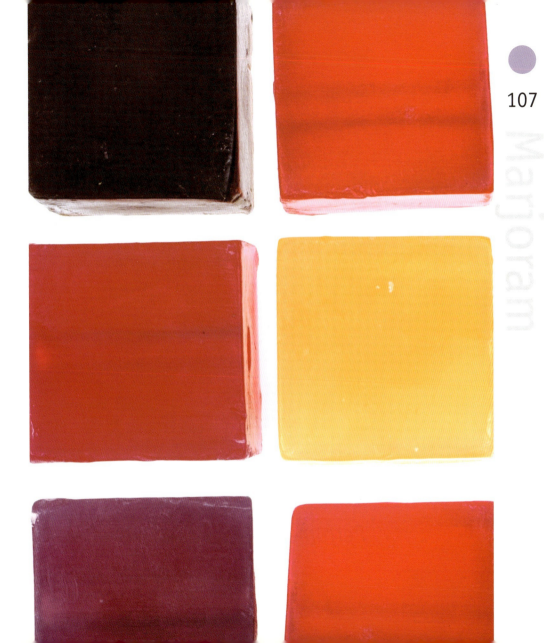

Marjoram

Myrrh

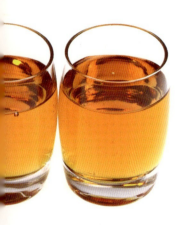

Myrrh

WARNING!
Do NOT use if you are pregnant.

Plant: Myrrh

Botanical name: Commiphora myrrha

Origins: Extracted from the gum resin of the bark stem.

Aroma: Smoky and balsamic.

Properties: Anti-inflammatory, antiseptic, and sedative.

Uses: This is excellent for healing wounds, and in caring for cracked skin and scars.

Suggested Blends: Cedarwood, frankincense, lemongrass, and patchouli.

Perfume Note: Base

Myrrh

Niaouli

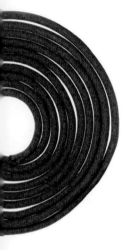

Niaouli

Plant: Niaouli

Botanical name: Melaleuca viridiflora

Origins: Extracted from the young twigs and leaves of the tree.

Aroma: Strong and camphoraceous.

Properties: Antiseptic and digestive.

Uses: For bronchial conditions and insect bites. This is a common ingredient in mouthwashes and toothpastes, and has been used to purify water.

Suggested Blends: Peppermint, juniper, and lavender.

Perfume Note: Middle

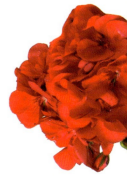

Plant: Palmarosa

Botanical name: Cymbopogon martini

Origins: Extracted from the fragrant grass, related to citronella and lemongrass.

Aroma: Geranium-like and sweet.

Properties: Antidepressant and a tonic.

Uses: Will alleviate nervous exhaustion and stress, and is also used to treat oily skin, acne, and dermatitis.

Suggested Blends: Cedarwood, lavender, and ylang ylang.

Perfume Note: Middle

Patchouli

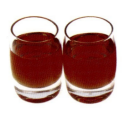

Patchouli

Plant: Patchouli

Botanical name: Pogostemon cablin

Origins: Distilled from the soft furry leaves which evoke the fragrance when rubbed.

Aroma: Earthy, musky, and improves with age.

Properties: Stimulant, antidepressant, and a tonic.

Uses: Used to treat dermatitis, abscesses, athlete's foot, nausea, and travel sickness.

Suggested Blends: Geranium, cedarwood, and tea tree.

Perfume Note: Base

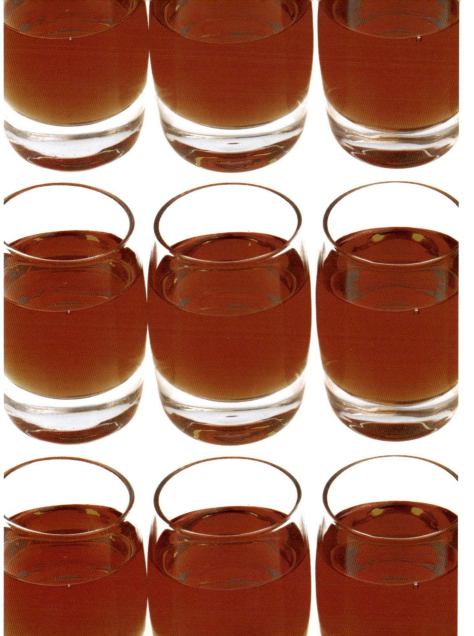

Patchouli

Petitgrain

Plant: Petitgrain

Botanical name: Citrus aurantium

Origins: Extracted from the leaves and twigs of the same tree which produces neroli oil.

Aroma: Bittersweet

Properties: Digestive and antiseptic.

Uses: This makes an excellent antidepressant, and is recommended for treating acne.

Suggested Blends: Clary sage, geranium, lavender, and rosemary.

Perfume Note: Top

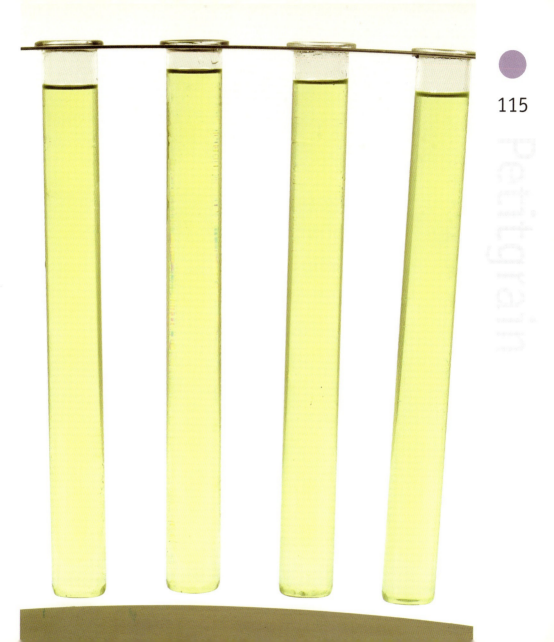

Petitgrain

Rosewood

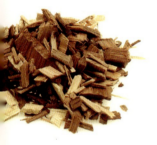

Rosewood

Plant: Rosewood

Botanical name: Aniba rosaeodora

Origins: Extracted from the chipping of the rosewood tree.

Aroma: Soft and woody.

Properties: Boosts the immune system and makes a good antidepressant.

Uses: Use this to rejuvenate mature skin. It also helps to prevent colds and flu.

Suggested Blends: Lavender, jasmine, tangerine, grapefruit, and lemon.

Perfume Note: Middle

117

Rosewood

Spearmint

Plant: Spearmint

Botanical name: Mentha spicata

Origins: Steam distilled from the flower tops.

Aroma: Warm, herbaceous, and mint-scented.

Properties: Digestive and a tonic.

Uses: A good treatment for headaches and nausea, and it is used in the treatment of dermatitis.

Suggested Blends: Tea tree, lavender, rosemary, and geranium.

Perfume Note: Top

Spearmint

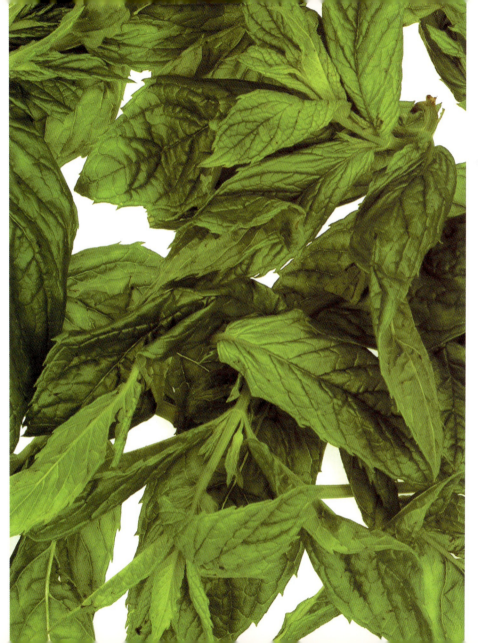

Spearmint

Tangerine

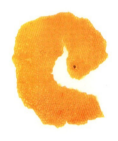

Tangerine

Plant: Tangerine

Botanical name: Citrus reticulata

Origins: Extracted from the peel of the fruit.

Aroma: Fruity and sweet.

Properties: Digestive

Uses: This is good for helping circulation, combating constipation, and diarrhea. It is also used to keep stretch marks at bay.

Suggested Blends: Orange and neroli.

Perfume Note: Top

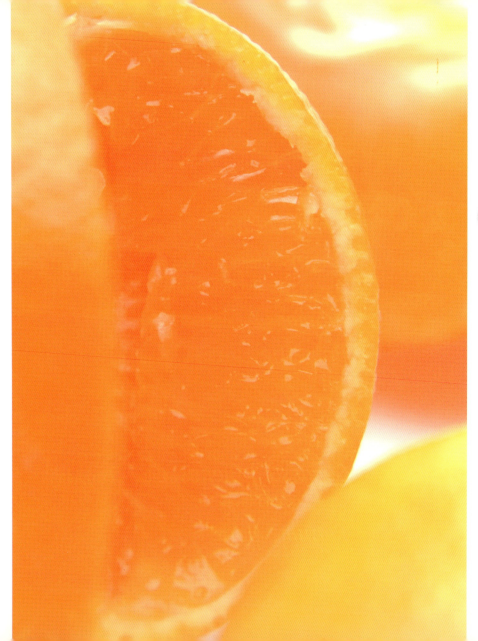

Tangerine

Thyme

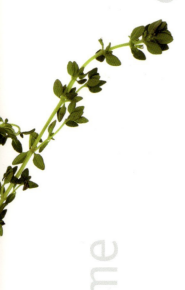

WARNING!
Do NOT use
if you are
pregnant.

Plant: Thyme

Botanical name: Thymus vulgaris

Origins: Steam distilled from fresh or partly dried leaves and flower tops.

Aroma: Spicy and herbaceous.

Properties: Antiseptic, diuretic, anti-rheumatic, and fungicidal.

Uses: Recommended for respiratory problems including bronchitis and asthma.

Suggested Blends: Lemon, marjoram, rosemary, and lavender.

Perfume Note: Middle

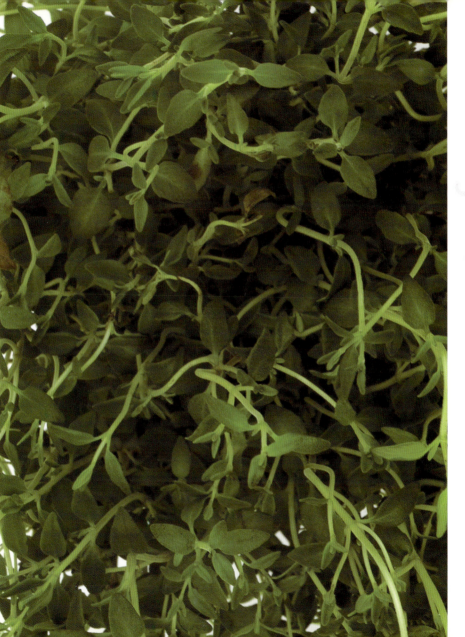

123

Vetiver

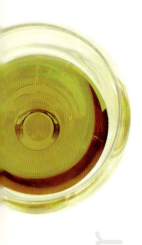

Vetiver

Plant: Vetiver

Botanical name: Vetiveria zizanioides

Origins: Related to palmarosa and lemon grass, vetiver is extracted from the dried and chopped (highly fragrant) roots of the grass plant

Aroma: Earthy and rich—improving with age.

Properties: The "oil of tranquility" is renowned for its calming effect and is a reputed aphrodisiac!

Uses: A popular fixative in the perfume industry.

Suggested Blends: Sandalwood, lavender, and ylang ylang.

Perfume Note: Base

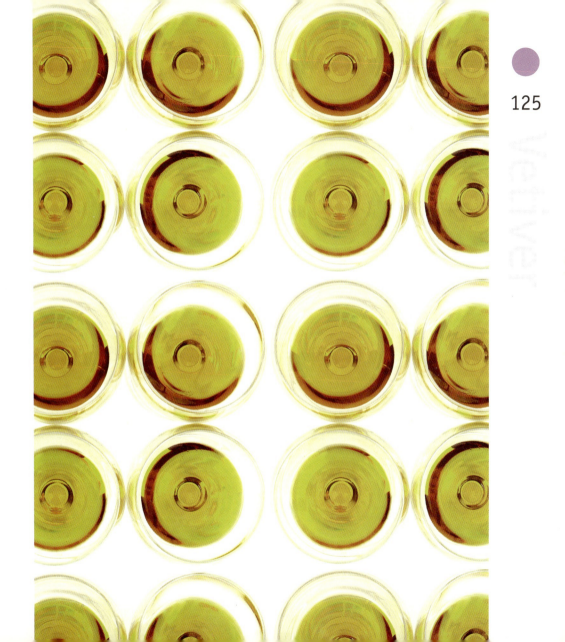

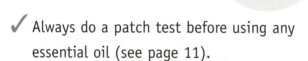

✓ **Dos &**

✓ Always do a patch test before using any essential oil (see page 11).

✓ Always dilute in a carrier oil before applying to your skin.

✓ Always keep essential oil away from your eyes and do not rub your eyes after handling them.

✓ If you are pregnant seek medical advice before using essential oils.

✓ If you are epileptic seek medical advice before using essential oils.

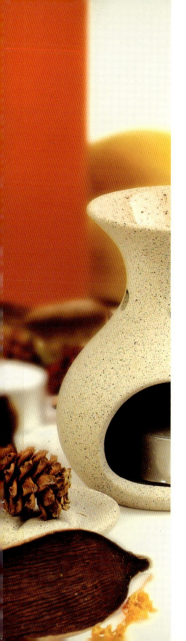

Don'ts ✗

✗ Never take essential oils by mouth, rectum or vagina unless medically instructed to do so.

✗ Never use citrus oils on the skin shortly before exposure to the sun. Citrus oils increase skin sensitivity to the sun and use may cause pigmentation.

✗ Avoid citrus oils if you have a history of melanoma.

✗ Never use an essential oil if you can find little information about it.

✗ Avoid prolonged use of the same essential oil.

✗ If you are asthmatic avoid steam inhalations.

Caring for your oils

Care for your essential oils and they will care for you!

- ✪ Essential oils are light sensitive so store them in dark glass bottles with stoppers.
- ✪ Store in a cool dark place.
- ✪ Keep out of reach of children.
- ✪ Do not keep oils in the bathroom where they will evaporate and become stale from the steam.
- ✪ Essential oils can last for up to 2 years if kept chilled.
- ✪ If you wish to keep them in the refrigerator, take them out an hour or so before using so that they will flow freely.
- ✪ Some essential oils improve with age— sandalwood, patchouli, and frankincense for instance.
- ✪ Essential oils in the citrus family last no longer than six months.

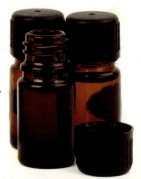